The Pre-Diet Plan

Everything You Must Do Before You Can Effectively Diet To Lose Weight

Dr. Sean Patterson, D.C.

www.DrPatterson.com

This book is dedicated to those who have spent most of their lives dieting, exercising and counting calories; those who have been given only small pieces of a larger truth, those who have been sold programs and potions that don't work, those who have endured a lifetime of dieting disappointment, this manual is for you.

Table of Contents

iv

Introduction: The Wedge

Have you ever felt as if a huge **wedge** somehow became jammed in between your efforts and your results? I want to take a moment to explain to you what that wedge is. Here is a mathematical explanation of why weight (fat) loss may have eluded you:

Large effort + ▼ (the *wedge*) = *small results*

Doesn't it make you angry? The **wedge** is blocking you from your goals. The Pre-Diet Plan will show you what your **wedge** looks like, and even better, how to remove it. So what is Your Wedge? It is simple; Your Wedge is Mis-Information.

Once that bad information is removed, things will look more like this:

small effort + **truthful information** = *large results*

You See, the Larger the Piece of Truth You Have In This Equation, the Larger the Result

Most people just keep increasing their effort thinking that if they just try that new diet or if they just push a little harder, then they will be rewarded. I know it sounds crazy that people

1

do this year after year, but it is true. I have even done it in the past. The reason is that the $60 Billion Dollar Weight Loss Industry is telling us mistruths, or to be fair maybe they are not mistruths, maybe they are just really small pieces of the truth. It is basically a lie by omission. An example is this- Everyone knows the best way to lose weight is to burn more calories than consumed right? Well that is partly true. It is technically not a false answer, but here is a larger piece of that truth: If your body is releasing certain stress hormones into the blood stream then you body will actually prefer to burn your muscle and bone for energy instead of fat no matter how little you eat. These same stress hormones will turn your exercise into a stressful event that will actually further break down muscle and bone, leaving you with a higher body fat than you started with. I'm sure you will find this sickening both physically and mentally.

Before we try to eliminate your *wedge (which means bad information)*, we feel the need to warn you about what is contained in this book. We want to apologize in advance for how rough the read (and the road) will be; nothing worthwhile in life comes easily.

So here you go:

The 'Pre-Diet' Plan (*Version 1*)

For many people, what we are putting forth in this manual may seem too good to be true, and will be dismissed as "cute but not effective." To that, we respond – "boo on you!" Why? Because this little guide can reveal the missing pieces of information to help you remove *your* **wedge** and bring you lasting results. The steps to follow are simple:

1. *Read a chapter out of the manual*

2. *Find a gem*

3. *Sit with your disbelief, skepticism or shock for a moment (a very briefly moment)*

4. *Now apply it to your daily routine*

5. *Begin to experience results*

6. *Repeat the first step until you are satisfied with your body and your health*

Not surprisingly, one of the nation's leading medical websites lists 96 diets whose titles are in alphabetical order (beginning with the Alkaline Diet, and ending with the Zone Diet) just to cover them all. We are not saying that these diets don't work. After all, if you don't know where you're going, any road will take you there. We're simply stating that they don't offer most individuals lasting results.

Our hope is that this manual helps you to gain more understanding of how your body works so you can get the results you seek. It's time to stop searching for magic pills, programs or potions once and for all.

Our goal is to help you spot dieting and weight loss fallacies from a mile away. While some people can starve themselves or even "over"-exercise off a few pounds, those who have done either can tell you that 99% of the time, the weight returns. We're not saying it isn't possible to lose weight and keep it off; we're just saying we rarely see lasting results. Over the years, having treated hundreds of individuals, we find that most people following prescribed diets and brutal exercise regimens lose a combination of water and muscle – not necessarily fat. Why? *Because a stressed-out body cannot and will not effectively burn fat.*

Long term stress cause the human frame to distort and become less functional. Most people's body distortions are a result of that stress. For that reason we have dedicated an entire chapter to the proper interpretation of stress. When stress is appropriately managed, fat loss can become a reality for people just like you.

For now, study the ***wedge*** model above and remember that failure to lose fat comes from a ***combination of stress and bad information, driving a wedge in between efforts and results.*** You simply can't remove this ***wedge*** by starving yourself, tricking your metabolism or over-exercising.

We believe we have created a roadmap for restoring your metabolism -- a GPS for your body. And we intend to give you all the "right" directions to your destination. To find out about regional or long distance speaking and consultation with Dr. Patterson, please visit TheRestoredBody.com.

Your scale: a BIG FAT LIAR
(Not all pounds are created equal ...)

Do you weigh yourself as often as you brush your teeth? Most people, who say they would like to be a few pounds lighter simply want to fit more comfortably into their clothes, feel better about the way they look at the pool, at a cocktail party, or a business event.

There is a difference, however, between *weight* loss and *fat* loss. During the course of our practice, we have worked with extremely heavy people with healthy body fat percentages as well as very light people who are, in fact, *fat*. Sound crazy?

That's why it's important to make a distinction between the number you see on the scale and how much of that weight is fat. *Body fat percentage* is defined as the ratio of fat weight to your overall weight. In my life, my body fat percentage has been as low as 7% and as high as 25%. That's correct -- I've been both a *heavy, thin person* and a *thin, heavy person*. Frankly, I prefer being right in the middle. My goal is to enjoy my meals while remaining able to see my toes (all of them, not just the big ones).

One of the best ways we have to evaluate body fat percentage in our office is to use a *Bio-Impedance Electrical Analysis* machine. We recommend that you find a health care practitioner who uses one, since it is considered an accurate test that offers extremely relevant data.

You see, simply weighing yourself on a scale cannot help you determine what is happening inside. If you see a few pounds disappear or reappear during that frequent check-in with your home scale, how will you know if you are losing or gaining fat, water or muscle? Because believe it or not, *it is entirely possible to lose weight and gain body fat percentage.*

We often have patients who gain a pound after their first month while following our recommendations. We get to watch them enter the office frustrated and dejected, and then watch that same person light up like a Christmas tree when their exam reveals that they've gained 6 pounds of muscle and lost 5 pounds of fat. Why? *Because under these circumstances, that one pound gain actually was an extremely healthy sign.* Who doesn't want to gain muscle and lose fat? For those of you saying "I don't care, I don't want to gain a single pound," pay attention here: Almost without fail, when your body fat percentage goes down, your body becomes less distorted and inches are lost.

Don't you care more about what you look like and how your clothes fit, than you do about the number staring back at you from your scale? Here is a riddle for you: You have a bag in each hand; one is filled with a pound of feathers and the other bag is filled with a pound of fat. You hold them up and drop them from the precisely the same height at the same time. Which one would hit the ground first? (Hint; remember that a pound is a pound).

We thought so. Like beauty, it's what's inside that counts.

How do your brain and body handle stress?

Some time back, a Harvard physiologist discovered that our brains are genetically hardwired to protect us from bodily harm. This response actually corresponds to an area of our brain called the hypothalamus, which—when stimulated—initiates a sequence of events that prepare our bodies for either fighting or escaping. The same is true when we experience excessive stress, whether from internal worry or external circumstance.

We were all bestowed with two adrenal glands, both of which sit atop of our Kidneys. These glands' primary role is to help us adapt to (and survive) stressful events; especially life-threatening events. Taking their cues from the pituitary gland, located in the brain, the adrenals know that when our brains signal an imminent threat, our *fight-or-flight* response takes over. But the brain can have a hard time differentiating real vs. perceived danger, initiating this response when we least expect it. An example? Have you ever been the passenger in a car when it appeared the car you were riding in was about to be hit by another car? What does your right foot do? Does it automatically act as if it were on the brake pedal itself? Does your body tense up? If the brain thinks danger is coming, it spins into fight-or-flight mode. Your foot is supposedly fighting what may come next, while your body is preparing for the worst.

Here are a few of the physical changes that occur when the fight-or-flight response is triggered.

- Blood pressure elevates

- Stress hormones such as epinephrine, adrenaline and cortisol are released

- Blood sugar goes up, which has a direct relationship to the amount of stress hormones that circulate through your body during times of stress

- Since your body is now in survival mode, it doesn't really care about digesting the sandwich you just ate, and blood is now directed away from your gut and redirected to the muscles and bloodstream

- Post Fight/Flight consequences include belly fat, bone loss & fatigue.

There are other kinds of dangers that will trigger fight-or-flight as well. Dangers unconsciously triggered in the brain are:

- Low blood sugar triggered by refined, high glycemic foods (these foods turns from carbohydrate to blood sugar at a rapid rate)

- Emotional triggered from people pleasing and unconscious anger or rage

- Physical dangers like cell phone waves, toxins in the environment and sensitivities to chemicals in your food.

Because of our fast-paced lifestyle and culture, our brains perceive danger more often than we realize, putting us in a constant state of low level fight-or-flight (LLFF). But the biggest offender is HURRY. Rushing through meals, cramming more and more and more into a day, never-ending sports and activities in which families feel compelled to participate -- simply spoken, HURRY is killing us. It results in weight gain as well as a host of other health problems.

The health care industry is constantly trying to come up with slick solutions for our weight and health problems, while Americans are getting fatter, sicker and more worn out than ever. But the solution is not more diet books and pills. It's putting a halt to LLFF. The solution is to stop hurrying and worrying and start recovering.

Your body's inability to calm down and recover can be the demise of your health, wreaking havoc on your metabolism. This is a very important concept to grasp. Once you do, your goal should be to stop hurrying through life, creating time for food, family, reflection and relaxation.

Does It Pay to Slow Down?
How A European Man Taught Me To Be Thin

Sometimes life hands you one of those paradigm-shift moments that can affect the rest of your days. One such moment came when I traveled to Seville, Spain.

My travel partner and I were hungry. Most Spanish hotel breakfast consist of a chocolate croissant and a cappuccino, but that morning we wanted something with a little more substance, so we searched for and finally found a little cafe that offered bacon and eggs. For those of you who don't know, Spain is known for its 'jamon' (ham), so there was a reason we became primal in our hunt for protein. When the server came to our table, my friend Chris began to order in the typical American way – no small talk, no huge smile – just a matter-of-fact, "I'll have the eggs................"

But we were in Spain, and in Spain, things are different. Fernando, the server lifted up his right pointer finger as if to say "uno momento", and then just smiled. He paused for a moment (which to us felt like an eternity), took a breath and then said these two impactful words -- "good morning." We were taken aback (and just a little bit embarrassed), but realized at that point that we weren't dealing with a robot: we were talking to a human being who had a life outside the quaint café we had just wandered into.

Fernando went on to teach us many valuable lessons that week, since we sheepishly chose to return to the café (on best behavior) to see what more the morning could hold for us. It was as if we became Fernando's collective *Daniel Laruso*, while he acted as our *Mr. Miyagi* from the movie *The Karate Kid*. We learned that he had a college degree, owned no car, was very comfortable in his body and lived by this motto: *"If work gets in the way of your life, change your work."* Fernando waited tables because he enjoyed it and it afforded him a healthy and relaxed lifestyle – period. Simply stated; Fernando was not stressed out.

The reason I tell you this story is because through my experiences at a Spanish café, I have come to understand the connection between a low-stress life, and a healthy, good-looking body. It all starts with you, the decisions you make and the way you choose to view the rest of your life. And like Andy DuFresne, the character in *The Shawshank Redemption*, you can "get busy livin' or get busy dyin'." What will you choose?

The 10 Commandments of Eating

Eating Ergonomics may well be one of the most important concept in this manual. Now that you're learning about how your metabolism is working, let's equip you with some tools to do something to get it working properly.

It does no good to pontificate about why you are having metabolism issues unless we can give you tips on what you can DO (and what you shouldn't do) about them. How have we come up with many of these tips? We've learned by watching—watching and imitating healthy (mostly foreign) people.

So what about those people who seem to break all the rules and still appear healthier and more slender? After all, they may live off of gelato, cigarettes, and bread, sleeping during the day and staying up until the wee hours of the morning, enjoying their cultural night life. What gives? Here is what I learned from them -- truly is the solution for digesting your food properly, losing body fat and lowering stress. Practice these techniques and you will start to restore your body faster than you can say "cheeseburger."

The 10 Commandments of Eating Ergonomics:

1. Thou shalt not eat while driving. Pull over and park if you are going to eat in the car.

2. Thou shalt not stand while eating. You may sit down or recline while you eat, but please don't slouch.

3. Thou shalt dine with others who eat healthfully.

4. Thou shalt refrain from "over tasting" food while preparing it unless it is truly to test quality or readiness.

5. Thou shalt take three deep breaths before taking your first bite.

6. Thou shalt give thanks to both the higher power as well as the chef before you begin eating. Make it sweet, to the point, and sincere, showing true appreciation for the amazing and abundant foods we get to eat and for the effort it takes to make them presentable.

7. Thou shalt drink one glass of room temperature water before the meal and one glass of warm tea or warm water with lemon after the meal. This is akin to rinsing off a greasy plate. Try *not* to drink during the meal, and if you need to, drink only room-temperature water with lemon --- never ice water.

8. Thou shalt not watch television, mess with a computer, fiddle with a phone or operate an electronic gadget while eating. Classical Music is a nice touch in the background. No commercials.

9. Thou shalt allow 15-30 minutes to eat if eating alone and one hour if dining with friends and family. Those slender Europeans know better than most of us how eating is a social activity – not a task to be accomplished.

10. Thou shalt eat slowly. You will really appreciate both the food and the company more when you slow down.

Eating Ergonomics really do work, helping you to focus on your food intake while making eating a deliberate act of self-love.

It's not what you eat; *it's how you eat it*!

Are you truly the result of what you eat? Pretty much. It's true that every cell in your body is made from the food, air, water, bugs and toxins your system takes in. However, it's important to note a different perspective on how food is transformed into body parts.

Some people are able to gain more nourishment from a low-quality, refined, processed, previously-frozen, fast food chicken product than other folks get out of a free range, organic, well-loved, fresh piece of chicken. *Your body's ability to gain digest and utilize the nutrition from your food has everything to do with the physiological, emotional, and ergonomic state of affairs when you eat it.*

We are not saying that it doesn't matter what you eat. For many people trying to lose weight or get healthy, what they're eating is LESS important than how stressed they are *while* they're eating it. As we mentioned earlier, when your body is in a low-level-fight-or-flight mode, you blood is diverted *away* from your gut. In addition to your reduced gut function, your immune system isn't as effective either. Vital energy is diverted away from these organs so all energy can be used to get you out of danger. Sad to say, but you can eat the finest of foods and there will still be a good chance you may barely process nor gain any nutrition from it.

On the other hand, let's say you are on vacation having the time of your life and you decide to go to a fast food restaurant. You may actually gain more nutrition from a burger, fries and a shake than you did from your organic, free range meal that you were eating while you were stressed out. Doesn't if feel as if you can get away with so much more on vacation? Now you know why. This concept may seem hard to grasp, but I assure you that as you read through this manual, it will make more and more sense.

Stress has always been around us -- gravity, saber tooth cats, infectious disease -- but never has a human body had to defend itself against so MANY stressors. These stresses include:

- industrial toxins

- heavy metals

- prescription drugs

- radiation

- cell phone waves

- physical and stored emotional triggers

- food refinement and processing

- even politics...!

Stress is all around us, from gravity to emotions as we navigate through this 21st century North American culture. We are caught up in a culture that offers much in the way of choices, fun and comfort, but also in one that keeps most of us locked in a perpetual state of LLFF (low level fight or flight), and thought to be the <u>root of illness, body distortion and weight gain.</u>

We want you to have an accurate understanding of why your body has been distorting and why popular methods of weight loss have failed you. You may be wondering when we were going to dive into food, calories and exercise. Truth be told, none of them are as important as the truths you are discovering within these pages.

Is Exercise A Healthy Way To de-Stress?

Most exercise should be called stressor-*cise*.

I calculated that I've spent over 10,000 hours (that is about 425 days) in the gym over a --- period of time, some days taking up four hours at a stretch at my health club. Those hours included working out, people-watching, chatting, observing trainers, etc., and here is what I came up with:

- Most people's bodies look the same or even slightly heavier year after year.

- Most people (especially women) look more aged every year.

- Most people have nagging aches and pains that get worse.

- Most people leave the gym more self conscious than they entered.

Did I say *health* club? Don't get me wrong: I am NOT anti-gym, sports club or health club. There are definitely ways of avoiding damage while improving health; I just rarely see it.

The definition of exercise is physical or mental exertion. Personally speaking, I don't really like those words. If you are a professional athlete, exertion comes with the territory. However, if you are a regular human being like me, you need Healthy Body Motion (HBM). You are probably already too stressed, and more stress through exertion is NOT going to help you lose weight.

High intensity, anaerobic and resistance-style exercise can make you very athletic and can be enjoyable as well; in fact, free weights, resistance training machines, and classes that typically encourage your heart to jump out of your chest can make you feel almost superhuman. Unfortunately for most, that feeling is coming from unhealthy stress hormones. These hormones contribute to belly fat, insomnia, high blood pressure, and digestive problems.

While I don't like exercise, I do like HBM (Healthy Body Motion), which I define as motion that is unpredictable, varies your heart rate and allows for motion in different directions. HBM does not trigger a danger response in the brain. Here are my six favorite forms of HBM:

1. Sightseeing or traveling; did you ever notice nearly every castle or fortress in Europe has a daunting number of stairs leading up to the entrance?

2. Gardening; everything from moving rocks to digging post holes.

3. Hiking and walking (especially hills and trails)

4. Sex with spouse (yours only please)

5. House cleaning; if you think of it as HBM, then you may actually enjoy doing it

6. Dancing

The trick is making your HBM activity fun and adventurous. Think of it as a way to strengthen your body and lower stress at the same time. In the interests of HBM, I find walking every day for 30-60 minutes on an empty stomach. Doing this encourages better sleep and gives me some time to reflect on my day as well. Walking without noise in your ears is best, but if you must, I encourage you to make your audio choice narratives instead of music. Listen to educational and encouraging information that excludes news that can introduce negative thoughts; every once in awhile, however, it's good to walk in silence without any wires hanging out of your ears. Gentle yoga and light stretching after your walk is a good idea too. Treadmill? It's not really about walking; it's about being walked. With that being said, here and there is fine on a rainy day, but do try to get outside and walk in nature. Try to focus on your mind, body and spirit while you walk, and avoid multi-tasking! Multi-tasking is the root of many evils in the body (like low level fight or flight), and it will surely work against you.

No Guts- No Glory?

Everyone poops, but in my practice I have come to realize that most people don't poop well. How is that for an opening line?

As someone in the health and wellness field, I ask about people's digestive health as well as their mental, physical and emotional health. And when I hear about distressed bathroom time, I see it as red flag that you have been stuck in a low-level fight or flight for some time. The fact is, most people do not have good digestive health. Too slow and too backed up is normally what I hear, with an occasional, "I hardly make it to the bathroom" thrown in. One of the most important tips I can give you is to work with your natural practitioner to improve you gut health. I also recommend learning more about the benefits of raw and fermented foods. The Internet is now filled with a number of blogs and websites dedicated to educating people on the benefits of raw and fermented foods such as kombucha, homemade yogurt, kefir, and fermented vegetables.

But take heart: even the people who have good digestion work at staying regular; eating incredible amounts of fiber, magnesium, etc. while avoiding cow's milk, flour and processed foods. Strange thing is, when people make the switch to eat more healthily, they actually get constipated at first. When they were living off a diet consisting of sugar, caffeine and refined carbohydrate, the bowels were overactive due to stress. So when the digestive organs have to digest whole, fibrous foods, they can get pretty overwhelmed and sluggish.

Almost without fail, here is why you have to heal your gut before you can lose weight:

- The gut really is the brain's pharmacy. Many of the brain's neurotransmitters for pain control, sleep and well-being are made in the gut. I have observed that people with a poorly performing gut also have allergies, slow metabolism, insomnia, low energy and even depression.

- Much of the immune system's ability to function properly is coordinated in the digestive tract.

- Many hormones are broken down and converted in the gut.

So I have come up with an alternative to that old adage that *you are what you eat*. The truth of the matter is that *you are what you digest*. Because if all those healthy minerals, antioxidants, and vitamins are not breaking down and being absorbed, then they are unavailable for use to heal and restore your body. And like many cultures throughout history whose economies have not permitted research on what constitutes healthy eating, individuals can become both overfed and malnourished at the same time – something I unfortunately see every day right here in my practice.

Tricking yourself to sleep

With four small children (and a cat named Dexter) at home, an undisturbed night of sleep is a rarity in my home. During my wife's pregnancy she would gain the weight, and after the delivery I would gain the weight due to interrupted sleep. The body does some great fat-burning at night; therefore adequate sleep is crucial to your metabolism. Here are some safe tricks to achieve a better night's sleep:

Many of us have blood sugar (insulin resistance) problems, meaning we are not properly utilizing sugar. For some, this means certain types of food cravings; for others, it means they cannot hold enough stored sugar (called glycogen), forcing them to wake up when the liver runs out. This often happens around the same time of day or night, as if there were a clock attached to waking moments. Survey says: 2AM is the most popular among those I have worked with.

Low blood sugar can also trigger hot flashes, which is a common reason for wakeup for women. The simplest of advice I give is to try indulging in a little protein snack about thirty minutes before bedtime. Try several stalks of organic celery with two tablespoons (total) of nut butter slathered on it.

Electronic media in the bedroom? No; try to banish the TV, computer, iPad and cell phone from your room, because you don't want all that alternating current and those irritating waves bouncing off your own direct-current body all night. If you have an alarm clock or electric items on your nightstand, make sure it is not plugged in right behind your head while you sleep. We are more like a battery; we charge up and then wear down. The waves from phones, internet, computers, etc., on the other hand, *never* seem to wear out. It's also best to avoid even using the computer, TV, iPhone, or any other electronic gadgets close to bedtime too.

- Read a book instead. The most relaxing types may be biographies, spiritual or self-improvement varieties – not page turners that keep you riveted.

- If you catch your mind spinning while you are trying to fall asleep or if you wake up in the middle of the night thinking, the problem may be mental stress. When you become aware that you are trying to solve tomorrow's problems, today, it's vital that you take control. This phenomenon triggers much of the "low level fight or flight" we spoke about earlier. Over-thinking, analyzing and obsessing is a massive source of stress.

The definition of anxiety is "distress of the mind caused by fear". *When we are living in tomorrow, we are triggered by fears caused by what has transpired in the past, since that is what we already know. For that reason, our brains try to create a new scenario to protect us from walking through those troubles again.* The key is to stop trying to solve tomorrow's problems with today's grace. Concern is normal. Worry can rob us of our health. Once you get to tomorrow, the solution often presents itself *after* a good night's sleep. Let your brain do its job and figure out tomorrow when it actually *is* tomorrow. This simple paragraph is one of the most important concepts in this manual.

- There is a gland in the brain called the hypothalamus. This gland tells the pituitary gland what to do. The pituitary gland, tells the thyroid, adrenal glands and sex hormones what to do. Sometimes the hypothalamus tells the pituitary to tell the Adrenals to release a stress hormone called *cortisol.* If this happens at the wrong time, it causes you wake up. Normal cortisol becomes elevated when you normally get up and get going. This whole process is called Hypothalamic Pituitary Axis Dys-regulation or HTPA, a problem that can be often seen with salivary hormone testing.

- And last but not least, Healthy Body Motion (typically on an empty stomach) for thirty to sixty minutes every day will help you get to sleep and stay asleep.

Counting Calories- Eat Less And Exercise More- Right?

For so long, we have been told that the best way to lose weight is to eat less and exercise more. But unless you are a 20-year old college student, crash dieting and over-exercising carries high costs – costs such as decreased fat-burning capability, inhibition of the thyroid and along with it, psychological stress.

I have been working with patients that are trying to lose weight for a decade now and have yet to find a calorie-counting diet that actually works beyond just a few pounds or for more than a few months.

We each have a basal metabolic rate telling us how many calories we need to sustain our daily physiological functions and support our lean body mass made up of muscle, bone, internal organs and connective tissues. Most people who have dieted and counted calories report that they have lowered their calories below their basal metabolic rate, and they still can't seem to lose weight. I believe this is caused by too many stress hormones undoing their hard work. When your body is in a "low level fight-or-flight mode", it makes it nearly impossible to burn fat and if you do, you run the risk of burning lean body mass along with it.

A stressed body wants sugar as its primary fuel, not fat. Imagine that you are dieting, eating a mere 500 calories per day and your stressed-out body is breaking down muscle in order to get sugar. I tell my clients that people who have historically consumed lots of sugar, refined carbohydrate, juice, fruit or alcohol will usually lose some muscle mass over the first few weeks using my program because the brain is over-reacting to a lack of glucose. It takes a little time for the brain to realize that everything is as it should be and that it is perfectly acceptable for fat to be transformed into fuel. I have seen this process take as little as two days and as long as a month and is one of the main reasons that people can diet for weeks and see no decrease in fat loss.

Let's Talk Food

If you skipped right to this chapter, it could be because you consider food to make all the difference. And you would be partially correct, because you probably will not lose weight, restore your body and get well without quality nutrition. However, changing the food you eat will not be enough. For optimum success, you must eliminate the LLFF (low level fight/flight) response in your body. With that being said, let's talk food.

There is never going to be a "perfect" food choice. However, there are definitely good, better and best choices. First we must impress upon you that foods that are processed are not going to support your weight loss nor will they improve your health. If you must eat packaged foods, make sure you rule out the ones that list words that such as:

- *Processed*

- *Enriched*

- *Pasteurized*

- *GMO (genetically modified)*

- *Irradiated*

- *Treated*

- *Hydrogenated*

- *Homogenized*

- *(Most) Natural flavorings*

- *Food dyes with "#" signs*

Is Organic necessary? I love organic foods, but just because something is organic, doesn't mean than it's healthy. Organic sugar is, after all, still sugar. It's also safe to assume companies spend quite a bit of money to get their products officially labeled *Certified Organic.* Food without that label, however, may be just as high in quality. For example, I have gone and inspected the cows, conditions and passion an entire Placerville ranch that sells non-certified grass-fed beef and found it to be phenomenal. It never hurts to spend a little time investigating where your food comes from and how it is treated. If I had to choose between an animal that never sees daylight, lives off of a constant drip of food and drugs, and grows faster than it should versus a well cared for animal that frolics around a pasture, eats grass and is humanely treated, I'm going to go for the happy guy every time. Even if food science says that the protein is the same; my gut tells me it is not.

What to eat and what not to eat? I like simple, single-ingredient foods. Typically, if you mix a few single ingredient nutrients together you get healthy food. It's when you are mixing multinutrient ingredients together that you can foul things up. Example: How about a salad with lettuce, kale, garbanzo beans, tomatoes, a little tuna and maybe even add a little vinegar and sea salt? All of those nutrients had ONE ingredient. But take a pre-packaged salad "kit" that contains croutons and processed dressing and there may be up to twenty five ingredients – ingredients such as beans with added stabilizers, non-organic cheese produced by cows that were fed hormones and antibiotics, and Caesar dressing loaded with everything from high fructose corn syrup to MSG.

Simple foods are those found in their pristine, whole form. These gems carry Mother Nature's original packaging, such as fresh, whole, unpeeled organic apples instead of becoming pulp with an applesauce full of sugar, stabilizing chemicals, synthetic vitamins, packaged in cheap materials months before their distribution or purchase. Yes, you can find organic applesauce in a glass jar, but it would still complicate the naturally pristine version of an apple. And perhaps organic applesauce tastes good, but the simple apple is still better. The goal is to keep a HIGH percentage of your diet whole and unrefined. Also remember that foods that have been turned into flour are highly refined and not good for your gut. Your mantra should be to keep it simple. Make what you eat mostly plant based, mostly raw, mostly unrefined and mostly organic. This will definitely help your metabolism perform better.

If most people just ate like this, most people would be feel and look healthy:

- Loads of veggies

- Moderate legumes (beans), olives, nuts and seeds

- Low (0-2 daily for most) Grains, Fruits and Refined Oils (cooking only with high temp fats like coconut and butter) Remember that olive oil is great raw, but heat can make it toxic

- Almost No sugar, juice and lab created foods.

- Stop Drinking Calories! This creates some of the fastest weight loss I have ever seen! When kids and adults reduce Milk, Alcohol, Juice, Creamers the results are incredible.

Oddly enough, a great way to consume more veggies while throwing out fewer rotten veggies is to *never place produce in refrigerator drawers intended for produce.* We all know how frustrating it is to pull outdated, rotting vegetables and fruits out of those drawers only to fine gunk and at the bottom of them. Put your produce at eye level instead, using refrigerator drawers only for food that does not spoil quickly. Instead of your eyes falling on all the meat, dairy and bread, you'll see lettuce, avocado, tomato, artichoke and even some apples. Good plan?

Here are some simple information about the foods for which people seem to be the most curious:

Fruit

Metaphorically speaking, the best fruit is low-lying fruit. What does that mean? From a literal perspective, most fruit should be treated like a desert. Go easy on it. One to two servings per day is usually enough. Stick to organic apples and organic berries instead of the more sugary varieties such as bananas, mangos, and oranges. Less is better when trying to lose weight. Did you know that the sugar in fruit, called fructose, is almost as difficult for the liver to process as the type of alcohol found in beer, wine and spirits? I see the best results when people stick to apple, pear, and some varieties of berries, all fresh and all organic. Lastly, make sure you *never* start the day with fruit or fruit juice, since it can cause a spike in blood glucose, causing you to have late afternoon crash. When your blood sugar fluctuates, it is extremely difficult to control cravings. Most feel better eating fruit by itself or with a little nut butter on it.

Dairy

I have no problem with dairy, but please make sure it is organic or that you know its place of origin. If you are healthy enough, you can drink modest amounts of raw, unpasteurized milk. Yes, I said *raw* milk. It's not uncommon for people with digestive stress, allergies or weight issues to improve quickly when eliminating pasteurized, homogenized cow's milk. Keep in mind milk is for babies- you ever see how fast a baby cow grows? I love whole milk plain yogurt with stevia to sweeten. I throw in a little cinnamon and raw pecans and that is my go to for breakfast and often desert. YES! I said whole milk plain yogurt. You see, "fat is where its at"! That is where all the fat soluble vitamins from the earth come from. Cow or goat eats grass that is deeply rooted—Fat soluble vitamins go from grass to animal's milk—you get the goodness. The "fat free" craze of the 90's only proved to make more Americans sick and fat. This is a whole different conversation, but remember this: Fat doesn't make us fat.....sugar does.

Vegetables

Cruciferous veggies rule, since they have great liver enhancing properties. Included in this veggie classification are broccoli, cauliflower, cabbage and kale. It's also wise to cycle vegetables as the seasons change, while trying to eat as many of them in the rawest form possible. Heating up vegetables can damage enzymes and alter the chemical nature of them. And don't fall into the trap of eating the same thing every day. Even if you love raw spinach, too much of it on a daily basis can contribute to problems with calcium, kidney stones and even constipation.

Animal Protein

We eat way too much animal protein. Some pretty amazing doctors and researchers are now starting to think excess animal protein is a leading cause of heart disease, clogged arteries and tumor formation. But eaten in moderation, animal proteins can be a part of a healthy diet. Try to keep your intake to no more than thirty grams of animal protein per day. This can consist of a few couple organic eggs in the morning and a nice little fist-sized chunk of grass fed beef in the evening. I would advise not eating too much high protein low fat animal protein, however. I think if you're going to eat the critter, eat the whole critter, especially the fattier cuts. "Fat's where It's at" when it comes to animal protein, assuming it is organic and grass fed. The hard to get vitamin and minerals will come up from the earth, into the grass, into the animal and into a body that is literally dying to get these nutrients. My opinion is that you should eat as little grain fed animal protein as possible.

Low Carb Diets

Most people who follow low carbohydrate diets end up consuming too much animal protein. Something seems to have gotten lost in translation, since many low carb diet books typically don't call for so much protein. Perhaps it's because animal protein is easy to come by and filling that it gets over consumed. Historically, it was the affluent or powerful people of the world who ate meat, while peasants ate beans and whole grains. Isn't it ironic, then, that the world's affluent tended to be plumper and sicker, while the peasants typically went through life with leaner, stronger bodies? Some very well respected nutrition authorities are claiming that excess animal protein can be responsible for higher formation of tumors. Most people I have consulted with report feeling great from 50-75 grams of animal protein per day (of course there are exceptions to the rule and this is an important topic to discuss with your natural health doctor).

Grains

Grains have created lots of controversy over the past ten years. Here is my take on grains- enjoy them here and there, but not more than once or twice a day. I enjoy grains in their whole form, or as close as possible. Steel Cut Oats and Brown Rice are among my favorites. I used to call Quinoa a grain, until it was pointed out to me that it was a seed- eat up! It is terrific from a nutrition point of view. IMPORTANT: I am not a big fan of wheat products and find that almost all of my patients lose weight and feel better when they eliminate them. Over the years, the size of the protein in the wheat (gluten) has gotten larger and harder to digest. I think it is worth your time to consider gluten sensitivity testing. This is best performed through stool testing. It will look for antibodies, sensitivities and more. It can have a dramatic impact on your health if you suffer from gluten sensitivity or celiac disease, so please consider elimination and testing.

Plant Protein

Vegetable protein is less efficient than animal protein. This means you will lose energy in the form of heat, which actually has a *good* effect on the metabolism. Among the best types of vegetable proteins are those found in legumes, such as beans. If you fear the consequences of consuming beans, be sure to soak them well. Legumes have always been God's gift to the peasants of the world, keeping them strong, healthy and nourished. We are blessed that we get to enjoy them as well. The protein found in legumes differs from animal-based protein, the excess of which the body will automatically want to STORE as FAT.

High Protein Eating Plans

Don't go there.

Alcohol & Coffee

Alcohol may be good for temporarily easing life's worries, but it's much better suited for sterilizing wounds. Although there are some health benefits to a glass of red wine, ingesting more than two or three alcoholic drinks per week will typically wreak havoc on your metabolism. Alcohol has a one-track metabolic pathway. If you don't need the calories at any given moment, the body will quickly and simply slam it into your fat locker. I love coffee! I use organics which have fewer chemicals, and I almost always mix my beans before grinding to lower the caffeine. I like a 3:1 ratio of decaf to caffeinated. Of course for most decaffeinated coffee is BEST, but I'm just being honest.............. A friend of mine refers to coffee as the nectar of the gods. He may be correct!

Here are some samples of my favorite, popular, healthy meals:

I like the idea of 4 meals per day.........with a couple of them being more like large snacks vs. meals

Early Breakfast:

Organic coffee with an egg or two (always the whole thing- not just the white), or an Americano with some whole milk plain yogurt with raw pecans/walnuts, complimented with cinnamon and sweetened with stevia can get your day going somewhere around 7 AM. Wait an hour and go on your walk.

Late Breakfast:

After your walk and if your schedule permits, try a late breakfast around 9 AM. Start with a bed of raw, diced cabbage, add warmed lentils and top them with an easy egg, If you're feeling frisky, top it with guacamole and hot sauce. Too complicated for you? If you don't feel like going to all that trouble, simply grab an apple and slop some nut butter on each slice.

Lunch:

If you want to go vegetarian during the day to keep your energy high try a vegetarian burrito bowl, consisting of beans, little to no rice, veggies, salsa and guacamole. If packing your lunch, bring a large salad loaded with beans, veggies, and maybe a bit of avocado or feta cheese. Broccoli with hummus is a good option too. And watch the garlic if you have to go back to work.

Dinner:

Try a small portion of animal protein like free range organic chicken thighs (notice I like full fat animal protein), a veggie (like asparagus or an artichoke) and a salad at dinner and exclude the grain if your goal is fat loss, replacing it with a second veggie. Another great meal is a beet salad, an artichoke with a dipping sauce made of garlic, olive oil, sea salt, pepper and maybe a touch of balsamic vinegar, accompanied by a fist-sized grass-fed rib eye steak or salmon on a cedar plank.

Dessert

Although you may dream of living off dark chocolate gelatos, doing so won't help you achieve your fat loss plans. So try to settle for a bowl of frozen berries instead. Choosing the frozen variety will stretch out the experience a bit, since they typically takes take longer to eat. By the time you're done, your brain will register the sugar and it will be much easier to manage your sweet tooth. For an extra special treat, make whipped cream using organic heavy cream, and add vanilla and stevia. It makes a great topping to sliced organic strawberries. Just don't do this daily...

A word to the wise: Even a high quality cheeseburger or pizza is junk and fast food should rarely be an option.

Non-Food Items

Some items found in food aisles can be classified as food, but should be avoided at all costs, since they can foul up the brain, endocrine system and damage metabolism in ways that are still being discovered:

- Partially or fully hydrogenated oils

- Food colorings that contain numbers Gluten

- BHT

- TBHQ (this can also be a preservative in lighter fluid)

- Monosodium Glutamate (and all things that contain *glutam*), saccharine, acesulphame, and aspartame.

These are only a few of the toxins hiding in foods that require label-reading vigilance on your part. Chances are that where you find one of these names I listed you will find all its relatives as well. To get an even more complete picture, simply type "dangerous food additives" in to any search engine and gaze at the formidable list of processed foods.

A final note: Beware of undiscovered food allergies that may be wreaking havoc with your metabolism. Even people who claim to have no allergies report they feel remarkably better when they eliminate wheat, corn, soy and cow's milk even for a week and often lose weight in the process.

The Inside Scoop: Techniques and Tricks

Now that you're on track, let's talk about some techniques and tricks that may help put your fat loss efforts on the fast track. Here are some ideas:

- Take pictures of your food and drink before you consume it. There is actually an iPhone application for this. Research has revealed that when you take a picture of your food before you eat it, you can actually alter your eating behaviors by making you reflect on and perhaps even reconsider what you are eating. It also enables you to share your food choices and intake with your accountability partner or health practitioner.

- Keep a written or typed food journal. Just as important as documenting what you are eat, is taking note of your state of mind each time you eat by asking yourself:

  (1) How do I feel emotionally? (Fatigue/stressed/fearful/angry/depressed)

  (2) Do I have physical pain anywhere in my body?

45

(3) Have I gone to the bathroom today? What was the nature and outcome of that visit?

(4) Am I clear-headed or foggy in my thinking?

(5) Am I experiencing any cravings? If so, what am I specifically dying to eat?

(6) Did I spring out of bed, or did my dog drag me out of bed? Am I eager to go for a walk, or would I rather head to my family room sofa, cover myself up with a throw and snooze a bit longer?

Your honest answers to these six questions will help you and your natural health care professional recognize patterns, assess and re-engage your motivation and aid you in changing course wherever necessary in order to achieve your fat loss goals.

There are no shortcuts to healing your metabolism. Please start to incorporate the instructions in this manual to the best of your ability. Whether baby steps or big leaps, just do it. No matter which diet, pill, program, practice or practitioner you utilize to get in shape or to get healthy, all of them will work a great deal better AFTER the ideas in this manual begin to soak in. And please do not attempt perfection. I go by the adage that perfection is the enemy of excellence. So strive for excellence!

Pills and Potions and Lotions – Oh My!

Pills, potions and lotions should be resorted to only when there is a true deficiency or when food and lifestyle alone are not resulting in meaningful progress.

As many of your know, we are fans of adrenal hormone testing through saliva. Think of it as a way to prove or disprove that you have been living in a low-level fight-or-flight. Saliva testing gives a snapshot of how your body handles stress, but please note that all labs and testing methods are not created equal. And while I like the idea of using natural hormones I am leery of patients (mostly women) coming in that have been slathering creams and lotions on themselves. This practice can prove disastrous and may lead to or contribute to ill health. Used appropriately and conservatively, however, these natural potions and lotions can reverse the signs of aging and prevent or even reverse disease. So our advice is to have your natural health care provider monitor the use of them.

Although I am a strong proponent of health and nutrition stores and natural remedies, be careful of ads that make claims about the powerfully speedy healing benefits of a magic berry that only grows in Antarctica and only produces fruit on February 29th of each year. Amazingly enough, when you reach the health food store – no matter what time of year – it's always on sale. It is important to consult with a natural health care professional when decided what natural supplements are good for you. People tend to *over-utilize* supplements, thinking they are some kind of magic elixir or shortcut and *under-utilize* the medicinal properties of food. We ask that you bring your bag of bag of supplements with you to your very first visit to us. Believe it or not, we have seen everything from a typical lunch bag-sized supply of supplements, to an overflowing handled grocery bag brought into our offices and our hearts go out to you, wondering how much you may have invested in all these pills, potions and lotions.

Here, then, is a road map of how we approach the use of pills, potions and lotions:

(1) Consult a qualified, referred health care professional.

(2) As a starting point, have bio-electric impedance testing done to see what forces are at work inside you.

(3) Alter your lifestyle; for every one or two positive choices you make, eliminate one or two unhealthy choices you have been making. An example would be to improve digestion, bone health and metabolism by adding daily raw broccoli

to your diet while discontinuing the glass of pasteurized, homogenized cow's milk before bedtime.

(4) Add supplements if deficiencies exist or they are applicable to healing.

(5) Begin to use natural hormones only after you have exhausted everything else in this manual.

If you are on the right path to restoring your metabolism, then you should begin to see changes within the first few of weeks. Some may be subtle and others quite overt. Look for improvements sleep patterns, measurable body inches, energy, occurrences of cravings, and quality of digestion, mood and memory. As for your scale, think of it as one of the least accurate ways to monitor this process, since your body will be adjusting to all these changes and fighting them at first. Stay the path, keep your motivation high and you can't go wrong!

Who Is The Man Behind the Curtain?

I am an 'Oh doctor.' How did I get the title? Because when someone asks me, "What do you do?" I take a deep breath, inform his or her that I am a chiropractor and the response much of the time is, "Ohhhh".

My schooling grants me a D.C. (Doctor of Chiropractic) and here in California I am even referred to as a Chiropractic Physician. I take that title seriously, because not only do I work with brains, nerves, bones, joints, muscles and ligaments; I also deal with physiology, anatomy, pathology, microbiology, embryology, biochemistry, nutrition, and sexuality, among several more *'ologies and 'alities*. I have been a student of health for most of my life, and my passion for it is still off the charts.

My practice began more than ten years ago in the form of sound chiropractic care to people who, to my delight, would become loyal and enthusiastic patients. Since then, my practice has evolved to offer so much more than simple chiropractic, however. Often, very sick people come to me with some chronic sort of illness or symptom, looking for a path to weight loss that could enhance their metabolism as they improve their health.

Weight loss is an obsession in this country, with people going to inordinate lengths to trim down. It's unfortunate, but I sometimes think a number of individuals would surely give up a finger or two if they could be guaranteed 10-20 pounds of weight loss. Where does this obsession originate? The quest for self-acceptance runs deep. What many of you many not know; however is that I have been where many of you already are. As a teenager, I was obese, weighing in at 200 lbs. at a height of only 5' 3." My nickname was "butterball" – not exactly the moniker the ladies are drawn to. Then I lost 60 pounds in six months and my life changed dramatically. Despite how much more attention I got from the opposite sex, however, the methods I used to drop all this weight damaged my metabolism greatly. As recently as a few years ago, I lost 30 pounds in only three weeks. That, too, has had its consequences.

You see, I put myself out there as a dieting and fitness guinea pig, having experienced just about every kind of diet on the planet partnering with crazy, trusting friends along the way. But I also found that the big business that propels weight loss in this country leaves most people wanting. After all, if everyone lost all the fat they needed to, there would be no need for health clubs, fat camps, diet books, and diet pills. Therefore it's profitable for companies to offer you enough success to keep you just hopeful enough while not truly striving to help you accomplish your goals. I really hate that business model. I must be one of those weird health practitioners who look forward to the day you no longer need me except as a friend. Why? Because my big thrill is watching people transform their lives through fairly unconventional means by using methods that can stand the test of time. It's what gets me up in the morning.

We're not really talking about diets here. We're not even talking about being fit, since I'm not demanding some kind of brutal exercise routine. We're talking about preparing yourself for better health, which pretty naturally helps your body get to its own natural set point. Sounds weird, but I assure you it works. Once you finish this manual and follow its guidelines, you probably will have little need for a diet any longer.

Having traveled over 30,000 miles, having visited dozens of countries, and having observed and studied the health of people in more than 30 international cities, I still have no double-blind studies or fancy write ups to show you. No medical journals have published my stacks of patient testimonials.

What I do offer, however, is practical and effective -- simple, healthy truths that can set you free. I just want to reaffirm this to you: Weight loss, Fat Burning and just Feeling Great are within your grasp. It is not as easy as most will tell you, but when you get the right information into your hands, and align that with your best efforts- you will accomplish your goals.

Yours in Health,

Dr. Sean Patterson

P.S. To inquire about a workshop or personal evaluation for you, a loved one, your church, or your place of business, please visit TheRestoredBody.com or email

DrSeanPatterson@gmail.com.

P.S.S. For a limited time, Dr. Patterson has released a controversial report to the public addressing; stress, hormones and chronic pain. Claim your free copy at

www.SecretHormoneReport.com

Made in the USA
Columbia, SC
13 April 2023

14785379R00036